47 Alzheimer's Preventing Juice Recipes:

Naturally Lower the Risk of Alzheimer's disease without the use of Pills

By

Joe Correa CSN

COPYRIGHT

ACKNOWLEDGEMENTS

This book is dedicated to my friends and family that have had mild or serious illnesses so that you may find a solution and make the necessary changes in your life.

47 Alzheimer's Preventing Juice Recipes:

Naturally Lower the Risk of Alzheimer's disease without the use of Pills

By

Joe Correa CSN

CONTENTS

ABOUT THE AUTHOR

After years of Research, I honestly believe in the positive effects that proper nutrition can have over the body and mind. My knowledge and experience has helped me live healthier throughout the years and which I have shared with family and friends. The more you know about eating and drinking healthier, the sooner you will want to change your life and eating habits.

Nutrition is a key part in the process of being healthy and living longer so get started today. The first step is the most important and the most significant.

INTRODUCTION

47 Alzheimer's Preventing Juice Recipes: Naturally Lower the Risk of Alzheimer's disease without the use of Pills

By Joe Correa CSN

Alzheimer's disease is a disease that gradually destroys nerve cells and links between them. The greatest risk factor for this disease comes with age, the majority of people with Alzheimer's are 65 and older. However, I have to point out that it's not necessary to enter a certain age for the disease to develop. About 200,000 Americans under the age of 65 have what is known as "early-onset Alzheimer's".

Over time, the disease leads to communication and understanding difficulties, memory loss, and abnormal behavior including loss of interest and even aggression. Alzheimer's disease is an extremely serious disease and the sixth leading cause of death in the United States. This is why it's very important to recognize the symptoms without confusing them with a normal old age behavior.

Alzheimer's disease, unfortunately, doesn't have a cure. However, there are some treatments for the symptoms that will not stop but will slow down the disease from progressing and improve the quality of life.

The exact cause of Alzheimer's is still unknown, but statistics suggest that women are more exposed to this disease. Doctors believe that specific factors combined together can greatly increase the risks and lead to Alzheimer's disease. People suffering from arthritis, poor eye sight, weak bones, depression, and hypertension are more likely to develop this serious disease. Naturally, poor diet and lack of exercise can develop a fertile ground for Alzheimer's.

Processed foods with lots of sugar, lack of vitamins and minerals, and trans fats are some of the habits that have the ability to harm your body in ways you can't even imagine. These poor diet habits directly weaken the entire body reducing brain functions.

In order to prevent and reduce the risks of Alzheimer's disease, it's crucial to change your lifestyle and improve your diet. Brain-friendly foods like green leafy vegetables, nuts, berries, beans, whole grains, fish, and olive oil should be on your daily menu.

Having this in mind, I have created a beautiful collection of Alzheimer's disease preventing juice recipes that are based on fresh and healthy ingredients and will improve your overall health and brain function.

These juices were carefully chosen to provide all the nutrients your body needs every single day of the year. Furthermore, they are extremely delicious and very easy to prepare. Make sure to try them all!

47 ALZHEIMER'S PREVENTING JUICE RECIPES: NATURALLY LOWER THE RISK OF ALZHEIMER'S DISEASE WITHOUT THE USE OF PILLS

1.   Orange Mint Juice

Ingredients:

1 large orange, peeled

1 cup of fresh mint, torn

1 cup of cantaloupe, chopped

1 cup of blackberries

¼ tsp of cinnamon, ground

Preparation:

Peel the orange and divide into wedges. Cut each wedge in half and set aside.

Rinse the mint under cold running water and drain. Torn into small pieces and set aside.

Cut the cantaloupe in half. Scrape out the seeds and cut one large wedge. Peel and chop into small pieces. Fill the measuring cup and wrap the rest in a plastic foil. Refrigerate for later.

Place the blackberries in a colander and rinse well. Drain and set aside.

Now, combine orange, mint, cantaloupe, and blackberries in a juicer and process until juiced. Transfer to a serving glass and stir in the cinnamon.

Add some ice and serve immediately.

Nutrition information per serving: Kcal: 157, Protein: 5.9g, Carbs: 51.9g, Fats: 1.5g

2. Green Watermelon Ginger Juice

Ingredients:

1 cup of watermelon, diced

¼ tsp of ginger, ground

2 cups of Swiss chard, chopped

1 cup of pineapple, chunked

Preparation:

Cut the top of the watermelon. Cut lengthwise in half and then cut one large wedge. Peel it and cut into small cubes. Remove the seeds and fill the measuring cup. Wrap the rest in a plastic foil and refrigerate for later.

Wash the Swiss chard thoroughly under cold running water. Slightly drain and chop into small pieces. Set aside.

Cut the top of the pineapple and peel it using a sharp paring knife. Peel it all and cut into small pieces. Fill the measuring cup and set aside.

Now, combine watermelon, Swiss chard, and pineapple in a juicer and process until juiced. Transfer to a serving glass and stir in the ginger.

Add some ice and serve immediately.

Enjoy!

Nutrition information per serving: Kcal: 127, Protein: 3.1g, Carbs: 35.8g, Fats: 0.6g

3.   Blueberry Lime Juice

Ingredients:

1 cup of blueberries

1 whole lime, peeled

1 cup of pomegranate seeds

1 small Granny Smith's apple, cored

¼ tsp of ginger, ground

2 oz of water

Preparation:

Place the blueberries in a colander. Rinse well under cold running water and drain. Set aside.

Peel the lime and cut lengthwise in half. Set aside.

Cut the top of the pomegranate fruit using a sharp paring knife. Slice down to each of the white membranes inside of the fruit. Pop the seeds into a measuring cup and set aside.

Wash the apple and cut lengthwise in half. Remove the core and cut into bite-sized pieces and set aside.

Now, combine blueberries, lime, pomegranate seeds, and apple in a juicer and process until juiced. Transfer to a serving glass and stir in the ginger and water.

Refrigerate for 5 minutes before serving.

Enjoy!

Nutritional information per serving: Kcal: 206, Protein: 3.3g, Carbs: 61.1g, Fats: 1.8g

4. Brussels Sprout Leek Juice

Ingredients:

1 cup of Brussels sprouts

2 large leeks

½ tsp of fresh rosemary

1 large fennel bulb

Preparation:

Wash the Brussels sprouts and trim off the outer leaves. Cut into small pieces and set aside.

Wash the leeks and chop into small pieces. Set aside.

Wash the fennel bulb and trim off the wilted outer layers. Cut into small chunks and set aside.

Now, process Brussels sprouts, fennel, and leeks in a juicer. Transfer to serving glasses and sprinkle with finely chopped rosemary. You can add a dash of Himalayan salt to taste, but this is optional.

Enjoy!

Nutritional information per serving: Kcal: 165, Protein: 8.5g, Carbs: 50.1g, Fats: 1.3g

5.   Carrot Fennel Juice

Ingredients:

1 large carrot, sliced

1 cup of fennel, trimmed and chopped

1 cup of cauliflower, chopped

1 cup of parsnip, sliced

1 whole lime, peeled

Preparation:

Wash and peel the carrot and parsnip. Cut into thin slices and fill the measuring cups. Reserve the rest for later.

Trim off the fennel stalks and outer wilted layers. Wash and chop the fennel into bite-sized pieces. Fill the measuring cup and reserve the rest for later. Set aside.

Wash the cauliflower and trim off the outer leaves. Cut into small pieces and fill the measuring cup. Reserve the rest for later.

Peel the lime and cut lengthwise in half. Set aside.

Now, combine cauliflower, parsnip, carrot, fennel, and lime in a juicer. Process until well juiced.

Transfer to a serving glass and refrigerate for 5 minutes before serving.

Add some turmeric or ginger for some extra taste. However, it's optional.

Nutrition information per serving: Kcal: 141, Protein: 5.6g, Carbs: 46.2g, Fats: 1.1g

6.   Beet Lettuce Juice

Ingredients:

1 cup of beets, chopped

1 cup of red leaf lettuce, shredded

2 large tomatoes, peeled

1 cup of fennel, sliced

1 tbsp of fresh mint, chopped

½ tsp of ginger, ground

Preparation:

Wash the beets and trim off the green ends. Cut into small pieces and set aside.

Wash the lettuce thoroughly and torn with hands. Set aside.

Wash the tomatoes and place them in a bowl. Cut into quarters and reserve the juice while cutting.

Wash the fennel bulb and trim off the wilted outer layers. Cut into small chunks and set aside.

Now, combine beets, lettuce, tomatoes, fennel, and mint in a juicer and process until juiced.

Transfer to serving glasses and stir in the ginger.

Refrigerate for 15 minutes before serving.

Nutritional information per serving: Kcal: 111, Protein: 6.9g, Carbs: 34.8g, Fats: 1.2g

7.   Pumpkin Cucumber Juice

Ingredients:

1 cup of pumpkin, chopped

1 cup of cucumber, sliced

1 cup of butternut squash, cubed

¼ tsp of turmeric, ground

¼ tsp of salt

2 tbsp of water

Preparation:

Peel the pumpkin and cut lengthwise in half. Scoop out the seeds and cut into small cubes. Fill the measuring cup and reserve the rest in the refrigerator.

Wash the cucumber and cut into thin slices. Fill the measuring cup and reserve the rest in the refrigerator.

Cut the squash lengthwise in half. Using a teaspoon, scoop out the seeds and clean it inside. Peel and cut into small cubes. Fill the measuring cup and wrap the rest in a plastic foil and refrigerate.

Now, combine pumpkin, squash, and cucumber in a juicer and process until juiced. Transfer to a serving glass and stir in the turmeric, salt, and water.

Refrigerate for 5 minutes before serving.

Nutrition information per serving: Kcal: 73, Protein: 4.1g, Carbs: 19.3g, Fats: 0.9g

8.   Cilantro Basil Juice

Ingredients:

1 cup of cilantro, chopped

1 cup of fresh basil, torn

1 cup of cucumber, sliced

1 whole lime, peeled

1 medium-sized apple, cored

Preparation:

Wash the cilantro and torn into small pieces. Set aside.

Wash the basil thoroughly under cold running water. Drain and torn into small pieces. Set aside.

Wash the cucumber and cut into thin slices. Fill the measuring cup and reserve the rest for later. Set aside.

Peel the lime and cut lengthwise in half. Set aside.

Wash the apple and cut lengthwise in half. Remove the core and cut into bite-sized pieces. Set aside.

Now, combine cilantro, basil, cucumber, lime, and apple in a juicer and process until well juiced. Transfer to a serving glass and add some crushed ice.

Serve immediately.

Nutritional information per serving: Kcal: 109, Protein: 2.7g, Carbs: 31.9g, Fats: 0.7g

9. Spinach Fennel Juice

Ingredients:

1 cup of spinach, torn

1 cup of fennel, trimmed and chopped

2 large red bell peppers, seeds removed

1cup of cucumber, sliced

¼ tsp of salt

¼ tsp of cayenne pepper, ground

Preparation:

Rinse the spinach thoroughly under cold running water. Drain and torn into small pieces. Fill the measuring cup and reserve the rest in the refrigerator.

Trim off the fennel stalks and outer wilted layers. Wash and chop the fennel into bite-sized pieces. Fill the measuring cup and reserve the rest for later. Set aside.

Wash the bell peppers and cut each lengthwise in half. Remove the stem and seeds. Chop into small pieces and set aside.

Wash the cucumber and cut into thin slices. Fill the measuring cup and reserve the rest for later.

Now, combine bell peppers, fennel, spinach, and cucumber in a juicer and process until juiced. Transfer to a serving glass and stir in the salt and cayenne pepper.

Serve cold.

Nutrition information per serving: Kcal: 125, Protein: 10.6g, Carbs: 35.65g, Fats: 2.1g

10.   Broccoli Cabbage Juice

Ingredients:

1 cup of broccoli, chopped

1 cup of green cabbage

1 large cucumber

1 large lemon, peeled

1 tsp liquid honey

Preparation:

Wash the broccoli and trim off the outer wilted layers. Chop into small pieces and fill the measuring cup. Reserve the rest for later.

Wash the cabbage and spinach thoroughly and torn with hands. Set aside.

Wash the cucumber and cut into thick slices. Set aside.

Peel the lemon and cut lengthwise in half. Set aside.

Now, combine broccoli, cabbage, cucumber, and lemon in a juicer and process until well juiced.

Transfer to serving glasses and stir in the honey. Add some ice before serving.

Enjoy!

Nutritional information per serving: Kcal: 150, Protein: 8.8g, Carbs: 36.4g, Fats: 0.9g

11. Swiss Chard Carrot Juice

Ingredients:

1 cup of Swiss chard, torn

1 large carrot, peeled and sliced

1 large wedge of honeydew melon, peeled and cubed

1 cup of cucumber, sliced

1 small ginger knob, peeled

¼ tsp of turmeric, ground

2 oz of water

Preparation:

Rinse the Swiss chard thoroughly under cold running water. Drain and torn into small pieces. Set aside.

Wash and peel the carrot. Cut into thin slices and set aside.

Cut melon lengthwise in half. Scoop out the seeds and then wash. Cut one large wedge and peel it. Cut into small cubes and set aside.

Wash the cucumber and cut into thin slices. Fill the measuring cup and reserve the rest for later. Set aside.

Peel the ginger knob and cut into small pieces. Set aside.

Now, combine Swiss chard, carrot, melon, and cucumber in a juicer and process until juiced. Transfer to a serving glass and stir in the turmeric and water.

Refrigerate for 5 minutes before serving.

Nutrition information per serving: Kcal: 92, Protein: 2.6g, Carbs: 25.7g, Fats: 0.5g

12.   Spicy Lemon Apple Juice

Ingredients:

1 whole lemon, peeled

1 small Golden Delicious apple, cored

1 large carrot, sliced

1 cup of celery, chopped

¼ tsp turmeric, ground

¼ tsp ginger, ground

Preparation:

Peel the lemon and cut lengthwise in half. Set aside.

Wash the apple and cut in half. Remove the core and cut into bite-sized pieces. Set aside.

Wash and peel the carrot. Cut into small slices and set aside.

Wash the celery and cut into small pieces. Set aside.

Now, combine lemon, apple, carrot, and celery in a juicer and process until juiced. Transfer to a serving glass and stir in the water, turmeric, and ginger. If you like, add some crushed ice.

Serve immediately.

Nutrition information per serving: Kcal: 105, Protein: 2.4g, Carbs: 32.8g, Fats: 0.7g

13.   Orange Pomegranate Juice

Ingredients:

1 large orange, peeled

1 cup of pomegranate seeds

1 cup of watermelon, peeled and seeded

1 cup of Romaine lettuce, shredded

Preparation:

Peel the orange and divide into wedges. Set aside.

Cut the top of the pomegranate fruit using a sharp knife. Slice down to each of the white membranes inside of the fruit. Pop the seeds into a medium bowl.

Cut the watermelon lengthwise. For one cup, you will need about 1 large wedge. Peel and cut into chunks. Remove the seeds and set aside.

Wash the lettuce thoroughly. Roughly chop it using hands and add set aside.

Now, process orange, pomegranate seeds, watermelon, and lettuce in a juicer. Transfer to serving glasses and refrigerate before use.

Nutritional information per serving: Kcal: 142, Protein: 5.2g, Carbs: 44.8g, Fats: 1.5g

14.   Avocado Peach Juice

Ingredients:

1 cup of avocado, cubed

1 large peach, chopped

1 cup of strawberries, chopped

1 large Granny Smith's apple, cored

¼ tsp of cinnamon, ground

¼ tsp of ginger, ground

2 tsp of coconut water

Preparation:

Peel the avocado and cut in half. Remove the pit and cut into small cubes. Fill the measuring cup and reserve the rest for later.

Wash the peach and cut lengthwise in half. Remove the pit and cut into bite-sized pieces. Set aside.

Wash the strawberries and remove the stems. Cut into bite-sized pieces and fill the measuring cup. Reserve the rest for later.

Wash the apple and cut in half. Remove the core and chop into small pieces. Set aside.

Now, combine avocado, peach, strawberries, and apple in a juicer and process until juiced. Transfer to a serving glass and stir in the cinnamon, ginger, and coconut water.

Refrigerate for 15 minutes before serving.

Nutritional information per serving: Kcal: 386, Protein: 6.5g, Carbs: 68.6g, Fats: 23.2g

15.   Asparagus Collard Green Juice

Ingredients:

1 cup of asparagus, trimmed and chopped

1 cup of collard greens, torn

1 medium-sized tomato, chopped

1 cup of spinach, torn

¼ tsp salt

1 rosemary sprig

Preparation:

Wash the asparagus and trim off the woody ends. Cut into small pieces and fill the measuring cup. Set aside.

Combine collard greens and spinach in a large colander. Wash under cold running water and drain. Torn into small pieces and set aside.

Wash the tomato and place it in a small bowl. Cut into small pieces and reserve the tomato juice while cutting. Set aside.

Now, combine asparagus, collard greens, tomato, and spinach in a juicer and process until juiced. Transfer to a serving glass and stir in the reserve tomato juice and salt. Sprinkle with rosemary.

Serve immediately.

Nutritional information per serving: Kcal: 66, Protein: 11.2g, Carbs: 19.6g, Fats: 1.5g

16.   Cucumber Lemon Juice

Ingredients:

1 large cucumber, sliced

1 large lemon, peeled

1 cup of avocado, pitted and chopped

1 cup of fresh spinach, torn

1 large lime, peeled

1 small ginger knob, peeled

3 oz of water

Preparation:

Wash the cucumber and cut into thick slices. Set aside.

Peel the lemon and lime. Cut lengthwise in half and set aside.

Peel the avocado and cut in half. Remove the pit and chop into chunks. Set aside.

Wash the spinach thoroughly and torn with hands. Set aside.

Peel the ginger knob and set aside.

Now, combine avocado, cucumber, lemon, lime, spinach, and ginger in a juicer. Process until juiced and transfer to serving glasses. Stir in the water and refrigerate for 20 minutes before serving.

Enjoy!

Nutritional information per serving: Kcal: 269, Protein: 6.7g, Carbs: 35g, Fats: 22.6g

17.   Apple Asparagus Juice

Ingredients:

1 large green apple, cored

1 cup of fresh asparagus, trimmed

3 large oranges, peeled

¼ tsp of turmeric, ground

2 oz of water

Preparation:

Wash the apple and remove the core. Cut into bite-sized pieces and set aside.

Wash the asparagus thoroughly under cold running water and trim off the woody ends. Cut into small pieces and set aside.

Peel the oranges and divide into wedges. Set aside.

Now, combine apple, asparagus, and oranges in a juicer and process until juiced. Transfer to serving glasses and stir in the turmeric and water.

Refrigerate for 10 minutes before serving.

Nutritional information per serving: Kcal: 316, Protein: 9.1g, Carbs: 98.1g, Fats: 1.2g

18.   Watermelon Banana Juice

Ingredients:

1 large wedge of watermelon

1 large banana, sliced

1 cup of strawberries, chopped

2 whole plums, pitted

Preparation:

Cut the watermelon in half. Cut one large wedge and wrap the rest in a plastic foil and refrigerate. Peel the slice and cut into small cubes. Remove the pits and fill the measuring cup. Set aside.

Peel the banana and cut into thin slices. Set aside.

Wash the strawberries and remove the stems. Cut into small pieces and fill the measuring cup. Reserve the rest for in the refrigerator.

Wash the plums and cut into halves. Remove the pits and cut into small pieces. Set aside.

Now, combine strawberries, watermelon, banana, and plums in a juicer and process until juiced. Transfer to a serving glass and add some ice.

Serve immediately.

Nutritional information per serving: Kcal: 273, Protein: 5.1g, Carbs: 78.8g, Fats: 1.6g

19. Zucchini Celery Juice

Ingredients:

1 small zucchini, sliced

1 cup of celery, chopped

1 cup of avocado, cubed

3 large radishes, chopped

1 cup of cucumber, sliced

¼ tsp of salt

1 oz of water

Preparation:

Wash the zucchini and cut into thin slices. Set aside.

Wash the celery and chop it into bite-sized pieces. Set aside.

Wash the cucumber and cut into thin slices. Fill the measuring cup and reserve the rest for later. Set aside.

Now, combine zucchini, celery, avocado, radishes, and cucumber in a juicer and process until juiced. Transfer to a serving glass and stir in the salt and water.

Serve cold.

Nutrition information per serving: Kcal: 235, Protein: 5.6g, Carbs: 22.3g, Fats: 22.6g

20.   Brussels Sprout Zucchini Juice

Ingredients:

2 cups of Brussels sprouts, halved

1 small zucchini, chopped

1 cup of cucumber, sliced

2 large carrots, sliced

¼ tsp of turmeric, ground

Preparation:

Wash the Brussels sprouts and trim off the outer layers. Cut into halves and fill the measuring cups. Reserve the rest in the refrigerator.

Wash the zucchini and cut into thin slices. Set aside.

Wash the cucumber and cut into thin slices. Fill the measuring cup and reserve the rest for later.

Wash and peel the carrots. Cut into thin slices and set aside.

Now, combine Brussels sprouts, zucchini, radishes, cucumber, and carrots in a juicer and process until juiced.

Transfer to a serving glass and stir in the turmeric. Refrigerate for 15 minutes before serving.

Nutritional information per serving: Kcal: 118, Protein: 9.2g, Carbs: 35.7g, Fats: 1.3g

21.   Melon Raspberry Juice

Ingredients:

1 medium-sized wedge of honeydew melon

1 cup of raspberries

1 cup of spinach, chopped

1 small Golden Delicious apple, cored

¼ tsp of ginger, ground

Preparation:

Cut melon lengthwise in half. Scoop out the seeds and then wash the melon. Cut one wedge and peel it. Cut into bite-sized pieces and set aside. Reserve the rest in the refrigerator.

Place the raspberries in a colander and rinse well under cold running water. Drain and set aside.

Wash the spinach thoroughly under cold running water. Drain and chop into small pieces. Set aside.

Wash the apple and cut lengthwise in half. Remove the core and cut into bite-sized pieces. Set aside.

Now, combine melon, raspberries, spinach, and apple in a juicer and process until juiced. Transfer to a serving glass and stir in the ginger. Add some ice before serving.

Enjoy!

Nutritional information per serving: Kcal: 142, Protein: 4.5g, Carbs: 46.1g, Fats: 1.4g

22.   Peach Apple Juice

Ingredients:

1 large peach, pitted and chopped

1 medium-sized green apple, cored and chopped

1 cup of watermelon, cubed

1 small banana, chunked

¼ tsp of cinnamon, ground

Preparation:

Wash the peach and cut lengthwise in half. Remove the pit and chop into bite-sized pieces. Set aside.

Wash the apple and cut in half. Remove the core and cut into bite-sized pieces. Set aside.

Cut the watermelon in half. Cut one large wedge and wrap the rest in a plastic foil and refrigerate. Peel the slice and cut into small cubes. Remove the pits and fill the measuring cup. Set aside.

Peel the banana and cut into small chunks. Set aside.

Now, combine peach, apple, watermelon, and banana in a juicer and process until juiced. Transfer to a serving glass and stir in the cinnamon.

Add some ice and serve immediately!

Nutrition information per serving: Kcal: 260, Protein: 4.4g, Carbs: 73.9g, Fats: 1.3g

23.   Sweet Avocado Mint Juice

Ingredients:

1 cup of avocado, pitted

1 cup of fresh mint, chopped

1 cup of strawberries, chopped

1 large apple, cored

1 large lemon, peeled

1 large cucumber, sliced

1 tbsp of liquid honey

1 oz of water

Preparation:

Peel the avocado and cut lengthwise in half. Remove the pit and cut into chunks and fill the measuring cup. Reserve the rest for later.

Wash the mint thoroughly and torn with hands. Set aside.

Wash the strawberries and cut into small pieces. Set aside.

Wash the apple and cut in half. Remove the core and cut into bite-sized pieces. Set aside.

Peel the lemon and cut lengthwise in half. Set aside.

Wash the cucumber and cut into thin slices. Set aside.

Now, combine avocado, mint, strawberries, lemon, and cucumber in a juicer and process until juiced. Transfer to serving glasses and stir in the water and honey. Add some ice and serve immediately.

Nutritional information per serving: Kcal: 376, Protein: 8.1g, Carbs: 67.8g, Fats: 23.3g

24.   Beet Spinach Juice

Ingredients:

1 cup of beets, sliced

1 cup of fresh spinach, torn

1 large red bell pepper, chopped

1 cup of purple cabbage, chopped

3 cherry tomatoes, halved

¼ tsp of salt

Preparation:

Wash the beets and trim off the green parts. Peel and cut into thin slices and fill the measuring cup. Reserve the rest for later.

Wash the bell pepper and cut lengthwise in half. Remove the stem and seeds. Cut into small pieces and set aside.

Combine cabbage and spinach in a large colander. Rinse thoroughly under cold running water and drain. Torn into small pieces and set aside.

Wash the cherry tomatoes and remove the stems. Cut into halves and set aside.

Now, combine bell pepper, cabbage, beets, spinach, and tomatoes in a juicer and process until juiced. Transfer to a serving glass and stir in the salt.

Serve immediately.

Nutrition information per serving: Kcal: 134, Protein: 11.5g, Carbs: 39.1g, Fats: 1.8g

25.   Fennel Apple Juice

Ingredients:

1 cup of fennel, chopped

1 medium-sized Granny Smith's apple, cored

2 cups of broccoli, chopped

1 cup of fresh basil, chopped

1 oz of water

Preparation:

Trim off the fennel stalks and outer wilted layers. Wash and chop the fennel into bite-sized pieces. Fill the measuring cup and reserve the rest for later. Set aside.

Wash the apple and cut lengthwise in half. Remove the core and chop into small pieces. Set aside.

Wash the broccoli and trim off the outer leaves. Chop into small pieces and fill the measuring cup. Reserve the rest for later. Set aside.

Rinse the basil thoroughly under cold running water. Drain and torn into small pieces. Set aside.

Now, combine broccoli, fennel, apple, and basil in a juicer and process until juiced. Transfer to a serving glass and stir in the water.

Refrigerate for 10 minutes before serving.

Nutrition information per serving: Kcal: 140, Protein: 7.7g, Carbs: 41.8g, Fats: 1.3g

26.   Zucchini Turmeric Juice

Ingredients:

1 medium-sized zucchini, sliced

1 cup of purple cabbage, torn

1 cup of celery, chopped

1 cup of cucumber, sliced

¼ tsp of ginger, ground

¼ tsp of turmeric, ground

¼ tsp of salt

Preparation:

Wash the zucchini and cut into thin slices. Set aside.

Rinse the purple cabbage under cold running water. Drain and torn into small pieces and set aside.

Wash the celery and chop into bite-sized pieces. Set aside.

Wash the cucumber and cut into slices. Fill the measuring cup and reserve the rest for later.

Now, combine cabbage, zucchini, celery, and cucumber in a juicer and process until juiced. Transfer to a serving glass and stir in the ginger, turmeric, and salt.

Refrigerate for 10 minutes before serving.

Nutrition information per serving: Kcal: 62, Protein: 4.7g, Carbs: 17.5g, Fats: 1g

27. Cranberry Blackberry Juice

Ingredients:

1 cup of cranberries

1 cup of blackberries

1 cup of cantaloupe, diced

1 small Golden Delicious apple, cored

¼ tsp of cinnamon, ground

¼ tsp of ginger, ground

Preparation:

Combine cranberries and blackberries in a large colander. Rinse well under cold running water and drain. Set aside.

Cut the cantaloupe in half. Scrape out the seeds and cut one large wedge. Peel and dice into small pieces. Fill the measuring cup and wrap the rest in a plastic foil. Refrigerate for later.

Wash the apple cut lengthwise in half. Remove the core and cut into bite-sized pieces. Set aside.

Now, combine cranberries, blackberries, cantaloupe, and apple in a juicer and process until well juiced. Transfer to a serving glass and stir in the cinnamon and ginger.

Add some crushed ice and serve immediately.

Enjoy!

Nutrition information per serving: Kcal: 169, Protein: 4.1g, Carbs: 56.3g, Fats: 1.3g

28.   Squash Plum Juice

Ingredients:

1 cup of butternut squash, cubed

2 whole plums, pitted and chopped

1 cup of strawberries, chopped

1 medium-sized apple, cored

¼ tsp of ginger, ground

¼ tsp of turmeric, ground

Preparation:

Peel the butternut squash and cut lengthwise in half. Scoop out the seeds and wash the both halves. Cut into small cubes and fill the measuring cup. Wrap the rest of the squash in a plastic foil and refrigerate for later.

Wash the plums and cut in half. Remove the pits and cut into bite-sized pieces. Set aside.

Wash the strawberries and remove the stems. Cut into bite-sized pieces and fill the measuring cup. Reserve the rest in the refrigerator. Set aside.

Wash the apple and cut lengthwise in half. Remove the core and cut into bite-sized pieces. Set aside.

Now, combine strawberries, butternut squash, plum, and apple in a juicer and process until well juiced. Transfer to a serving glass and add some crushed ice.

Serve immediately.

Nutrition information per serving: Kcal: 214, Protein: 4.1g, Carbs: 65.2g, Fats: 1.2g

29.   Orange Spinach Juice

Ingredients:

1 large orange, peeled

½ cup of spinach, torn

1 cup of pineapple, chunked

3 Brussels sprouts, halved

1 oz of water

1 tsp of liquid honey

Preparation:

Peel the orange and divide into wedges. Cut each wedge in half and set aside.

Wash the spinach thoroughly under cold running water and torn with hands. Set aside.

Using a sharp paring knife, cut the top of the pineapple. Gently remove all hard skin and slice it into thin slices. Fill the measuring cup and reserve the rest for later.

Wash the Brussels sprouts and trim off the wilted leaves. Cut each in half and set aside.

Now, combine pineapple, orange, spinach, and Brussels sprouts in a juicer and process until well juiced. Transfer to a serving glass and stir in the honey and water.

Refrigerate for 10 minutes before serving.

Enjoy!

Nutrition information per serving: Kcal: 172, Protein: 7.9g, Carbs: 52.7g, Fats: 1.1g

30.   Carrot Collard Green Juice

Ingredients:

1 large carrot, chopped

1 cup of collard greens, torn

1 cup of avocado, chunked

1 cup of Romaine lettuce, shredded

1 whole cucumber, sliced

¼ tsp of ginger, ground

Preparation:

Wash and peel the carrot. Cut into thin slices and set aside.

Combine collard greens and lettuce in a large colander. Wash thoroughly under cold running water. Drain and shred. Set aside.

Peel the avocado and cut lengthwise in half. Remove the pit and cut into small chunks. Fill the measuring cup and reserve the rest in the refrigerator.

Wash the cucumber and cut into thin slices. Fill the measuring cup and reserve the rest for later. Set aside.

Now, combine carrot, collard greens, avocado, lettuce, and cucumber in a juicer and process until juiced. Transfer to a serving glass and stir in the ginger.

Refrigerate for 5 minutes before serving.

Nutrition information per serving: Kcal: 271, Protein: 7.3g, Carbs: 34.1g, Fats: 22.8g

31.   Lemon Spinach Juice

Ingredients:

1 cup of sweet potato, cubed

1 whole lemon, peeled

1 cup of fresh spinach, torn

1 cup of pomegranate seeds

2 oz of water

Preparation:

Peel the lemon and cut lengthwise in half. Set aside.

Wash the spinach thoroughly under cold running water. Drain and torn into small pieces. Set aside.

Peel the sweet potato and cut into small cubes. Place in a deep pot and add 3 cups of water. Bring it to a boil and cook for 5 minutes. Remove from the heat and drain. Set aside.

Cut the top of the pomegranate fruit using a sharp paring knife. Slice down to each of the white membranes inside of the fruit. Pop the seeds into a measuring cup and set aside.

Now, combine lemon, spinach, previously cooked potato, and pomegranate seeds in a juicer. Process until well juiced.

Transfer to a serving glass and stir in the water. Add some ice and serve immediately.

Enjoy!

Nutritional information per serving: Kcal: 195, Protein: 10.2g, Carbs: 56.1g, Fats: 2.1g

32.   Mustard Green Parsley Juice

Ingredients:

1 cup of mustard greens, torn

1 cup of parsley, torn

2 cups of Romaine lettuce, chopped

1 medium-sized Roma tomato, chopped

1 whole cucumber, sliced

¼ tsp of turmeric, ground

¼ tsp of salt

Preparation:

Combine mustard greens and parsley in a large colander. Rinse well and drain. Torn into small pieces and set aside.

Rinse the lettuce thoroughly under cold running water. Chop into small pieces and set aside.

Wash the tomato and place in a bowl. Chop into bite-sized pieces and reserve the tomato juice while cutting. Set aside.

Wash the cucumber and cut into thin slices. Set aside.

Now, combine lettuce, tomato, mustard greens, parsley, and cucumber in a juicer and process until juiced. Transfer to a serving glass and stir in the turmeric, salt, and reserved tomato juice.

Serve cold.

Nutrition information per serving: Kcal: 85, Protein: 7.6g, Carbs: 25.3g, Fats: 1.6g

33.   Lime Papaya Juice

Ingredients:

1 large lime, peeled

1 small papaya, seeded and peeled

1 cup of strawberries

1 cup of cranberries

3 oz of coconut water

Preparation:

Peel the lime and cut lengthwise in half. Set aside.

Peel the papaya and cut lengthwise in half. Scoop out the black seeds and flesh using a spoon. Cut into small chunks and set aside.

Place the strawberries and cranberries in a colander and wash under cold running water. Drain and set aside.

Now, process papaya, lime, strawberries, and cranberries in a juicer. Transfer to serving glasses and stir in the coconut water.

Add some ice, or refrigerate for 10 minutes before serving.

Enjoy!

Nutritional information per serving: Kcal: 153, Protein: 2.6g, Carbs: 50.9g, Fats: 1.8g

34.   Apple Strawberry Juice

Ingredients:

1 large red apple, cored

2 large strawberries, chopped

2 large grapefruits, peeled

1 small ginger knob, peeled

2 oz of coconut water

Preparation:

Wash the apple and cut in half. Remove the core and cut into bite-sized pieces. Set aside.

Wash the strawberries and cut into small pieces. Set aside.

Peel the grapefruits and divide into wedges. Set aside.

Peel the ginger knob and set aside.

Now, combine grapefruits, apple, strawberries, and ginger in a juicer. Process until well juiced and transfer to serving glasses. Stir in the coconut water and refrigerate for 10 minutes before serving.

Enjoy!

Nutritional information per serving: Kcal: 302, Protein: 4.8g, Carbs: 86.3g, Fats: 1.7g

35.   Apple Potato Juice

Ingredients:

1 medium-sized Golden Delicious apple, cored

1 cup of sweet potatoes, cubed

1 cup of celery, chopped

1 medium-sized orange, peeled

1 tbsp of fresh mint, torn

Preparation:

Wash the apple and cut lengthwise in half. Remove the core and cut into bite-sized pieces. Set aside.

Peel the sweet potato and cut into small cubes. Fill the measuring cup and reserve the rest for later. Set aside.

Wash the celery and cut into bite-sized pieces. Set aside.

Peel the orange and divide into wedges. Cut each wedge in half and set aside.

Now, combine sweet potatoes, celery, apple, and orange in a juicer. Process until well juiced. Transfer to a serving glass and sprinkle with mint.

Add some crushed ice and serve immediately.

Nutrition information per serving: Kcal: 236, Protein: 4.7g, Carbs: 67.8g, Fats: 0.7g

36.   Zucchini Lemon Juice

Ingredients:

1 medium-sized zucchini, chopped

1 whole lemon, peeled

1 cup of fresh kale, chopped

1 whole lime, peeled

1 cup of fresh mint, torn

Preparation:

Wash the zucchini and cut into small pieces. Set aside.

Peel the lemon and lime. Cut lengthwise in half and set aside.

Rinse the kale thoroughly under cold running water. Drain and chop into small pieces. Set aside.

Wash the mint and chop into small pieces. Set aside.

Now, combine zucchini, lemon, kale, lime, and mint in a juicer. Process until well juiced. Transfer to a serving glass and add some crushed ice.

Serve immediately.

Nutrition information per serving: Kcal: 79, Protein: 7g, Carbs: 24.7g, Fats: 1.7g

37.   Cucumber Artichoke Juice

Ingredients:

1 large cucumber

1 large artichoke head

1 cup of turnip greens

5 large asparagus spears

¼ tsp of ginger, ground

1 oz of water

Preparation:

Wash the cucumber and cut into thick slices. Set aside.

Using a sharp knife, trim off the outer leave of the artichoke. Cut into small pieces and set aside.

Wash the turnip greens and roughly chop it using hands. Set aside.

Wash the asparagus spears and trim off the woody ends. Cut into small pieces and set aside.

Now, process turnip greens, cucumber, artichoke, and asparagus in a juicer.

Transfer to serving glasses and stir in the ginger and water.

Add few ice cubes before serving.

Nutritional information per serving: Kcal: 101, Protein: 10.1g, Carbs: 35.8g, Fats: 0.8g

38.   Cantaloupe Cucumber Juice

Ingredients:

1 cup of cantaloupe, peeled and chopped

1 large cucumber

1 cup of avocado, peeled and pitted

1 large lemon, peeled

Preparation:

Cut the cantaloupe in half. Scoop out the seeds and flesh. Cut two wedges and peel them. Chop into chunks and set aside. Reserve the rest of the cantaloupe in a refrigerator.

Wash the cucumber and cut into thick slices. Set aside.

Peel the avocado and cut in half. Remove the pit and cut into chunks. Set aside.

Peel the lemon and cut in half. Set aside.

Now, process cantaloupe, cucumber, avocado, and lemon in a juicer.

Transfer to serving glasses and add some water to adjust the thickness, if needed.

Add some ice and serve immediately.

Nutritional information per serving: Kcal: 292, Protein: 6.8g, Carbs: 41.5g, Fats: 22.2g

39.   Ginger Carrot Juice

Ingredients:

1 large carrot, sliced

1 cup of pumpkin, cubed

1 cup of cucumber, sliced

1 large orange, peeled and wedged

1 small ginger knob, chopped

Preparation:

Wash and peel the carrot. Cut into thin slices and set aside.

Cut the top of a pumpkin. Cut lengthwise in half and then scrape out the seeds. Cut one large wedge and peel it. Cut into small cubes and fill the measuring cup. Reserve the rest in the refrigerator.

Wash the cucumber and cut into thin slices. Fill the measuring cup and reserve the rest for later. Set aside.

Peel the orange and divide into wedges. Cut each wedge in half and set aside.

Peel the ginger knob and cut into small pieces. Set aside.

Now, combine pumpkin, carrot, cucumber, orange, and ginger in a juicer. Process until well juiced. Transfer to a serving glass and add some ice.

Serve immediately.

Nutrition information per serving: Kcal: 130, Protein: 4.1g, Carbs: 39.1g, Fats: 0.6g

40. Lettuce Cabbage Juice

Ingredients:

1 cup of red leaf lettuce, chopped

1 cup of purple cabbage, chopped

1 medium-sized artichoke, chopped

1 cup of fresh basil, torn

1 cup of cucumber, sliced

1 large carrot, sliced

Preparation:

Combine lettuce and cabbage in a large colander and rinse well under cold running water. Drain and chop into small pieces. Set aside.

Trim off the outer layers of the artichoke using a sharp paring knife. Cut into bite-sized pieces and set aside.

Rinse the basil with cold water and torn into small pieces. Set aside.

Wash the cucumber and cut into thin slices. Fill the measuring cup and reserve the rest in the refrigerator.

Wash and peel the carrot. Cut into thin slices and set aside.

Now, combine artichoke, basil, lettuce, cabbage, cucumber, and carrot in a juicer and process until juiced.

Transfer to a serving glass and serve immediately.

Nutritional information per serving: Kcal: 88, Protein: 7.6g, Carbs: 30.1g, Fats: 0.7g

41.   Basil Cucumber Juice

Ingredients:

1 cup of fresh basil, torn

1 cup of cucumber, sliced

1 medium-sized zucchini, chopped

1 cup of red leaf lettuce, torn

1 cup of avocado, cut into bite-sized pieces

Preparation:

Combine basil and lettuce in a large colander and rinse under cold running water. Drain and torn with hands into small pieces. Set aside.

Wash the cucumber and cut into thin slices. Fill the measuring cup and refrigerate for later.

Peel the zucchini and chop into small pieces. Set aside.

Peel the avocado and cut lengthwise in half. Remove the pit and cut into bite-sized pieces. Fill the measuring cup and reserve the rest in the refrigerator.

Now, combine zucchini, basil, lettuce, avocado, and cucumber in a juicer. Process until well juiced. Transfer to a serving glass and add some ice.

Serve immediately.

Nutrition information per serving: Kcal: 234, Protein: 6.7g, Carbs: 21.7g, Fats: 22.3g

42. Celery Leek Juice

Ingredients:

1 cup of celery, chopped

1 whole leek, chopped

2 cups of parsley, torn

1 whole cucumber, sliced

1 cup of beet greens, torn

¼ tsp of turmeric powder, ground

¼ tsp of cumin, ground

Preparation:

Wash the celery and chop into small pieces. Fill the measuring cup and reserve the rest in the refrigerator. Set aside.

Wash the leek and chop into bite-sized pieces. Set aside.

Combine parsley and beet greens in a large colander. Rinse well under cold running water and drain. Torn into small pieces and set aside.

Wash the cucumber and cut into thin slices. Set aside.

Now, combine celery, leek, parsley, beet greens, and cucumber in a juicer and process until juiced. Transfer to a serving glass and stir in the turmeric and cumin.

Serve immediately.

Nutrition information per serving: Kcal: 127, Protein: 8.4g, Carbs: 35.7g, Fats: 1.7g

43.   Cucumber Banana Juice

Ingredients:

1 cup of cucumber, sliced

1 medium-sized banana, sliced

1 small Granny Smith's apple, cored

1 tbsp of aloe juice

1 large celery stalk, chopped

Preparation:

Wash the cucumber and cut into thin slices. Fill the measuring cup and reserve the rest for later. Set aside.

Peel the banana and cut into chunks. Set aside.

Wash the apple and cut in half. Remove the core and cut into bite-sized pieces. Set aside.

Wash the celery stalk and chop into bite-sized pieces. Set aside.

Now, combine cucumber, banana, apple, and celery in a juicer. Process until juiced.

Transfer to a serving glass and stir in the aloe juice.

Add some crushed ice and serve immediately.

Nutrition information per serving: Kcal: 174, Protein: 2.7g, Carbs: 50.3g, Fats: 0.8g

44.   Onion Pepper Juice

Ingredients:

1 medium-sized spring onion

1 large bell pepper, seeded

1 cup of cherry tomatoes

1 garlic clove, peeled

¼ tsp of Cayenne pepper, ground

¼ tsp of salt

A handful of fresh cilantro

Preparation:

Wash the spring onion and chop into small pieces. Set aside.

Wash the bell pepper and cut in half. Remove the seeds and chop into small pieces. Set aside.

Wash the cherry tomatoes and place them in a bowl. Cut in half and reserve the juice while cutting. Set aside.

Peel the garlic and set aside.

Wash the cilantro thoroughly and torn with hands. Set aside.

Now, combine tomatoes, spring onion, cilantro, bell pepper, and garlic in a juicer and process until juiced.

Transfer to serving glasses and stir in Cayenne pepper and salt.

Refrigerate for 5 minutes and serve.

Nutritional information per serving: Kcal: 41, Protein: 2.8g, Carbs: 11.5g, Fats: 0.6g

45.   Celery Grapefruit Juice

Ingredients:

1 cup of celery, chopped

1 whole grapefruit, peeled

2 large carrots, chunked

1 small Golden Delicious apple, cored and chopped

¼ tsp of cinnamon, ground

Preparation:

Wash the celery and cut into small pieces. Fill the measuring cup and reserve the rest in the refrigerator.

Peel the grapefruit and divide into wedges. Cut each wedge in half and set aside.

Wash and peel the carrots. Cut into small chunks and set aside.

Wash the apple and cut lengthwise in half. Remove the core and cut into bite-sized pieces. Set aside.

Now, combine celery, grapefruit, carrots, and apple in a juicer and process until well juiced. Transfer to a serving glass and stir in the cinnamon.

Add some crushed ice and serve immediately.

Enjoy!

Nutritional information per serving: Kcal: 203, Protein: 4.3g, Carbs: 60.6g, Fats: 1.1g

46.   Plum Cantaloupe Juice

Ingredients:

1 whole plum, chopped

1 cup of cantaloupe, chopped

1 large orange, peeled

1 cup of fresh mint, torn

¼ tsp of turmeric, ground

¼ tsp of ginger, ground

Preparation:

Wash the plum and cut in half. Remove the pit and chop into small pieces. Set aside.

Cut the cantaloupe in half. Scoop out the seeds and flesh. Cut and peel one large wedge. Chop into chunks and fill the measuring cup. Reserve the rest of the cantaloupe in a refrigerator.

Peel the orange and divide into wedges. Cut each wedge in half and set aside.

Wash the mint thoroughly under cold running water. Torn into small pieces and set aside.

Now, combine plum, cantaloupe, orange, and mint in a juicer and process until juiced. Transfer to a serving glass and stir in the turmeric and ginger.

Add some ice and serve immediately.

Enjoy!

Nutritional information per serving: Kcal: 151, Protein: 4.4g, Carbs: 45.6g, Fats: 0.9g

47.   Apricot Swiss Chard Juice

Ingredients:

3 whole apricots, pitted

1 cup of Swiss chard, torn

1 whole grapefruit, peeled and wedged

1 medium-sized apple, cored

1 tbsp of liquid honey

¼ tsp of ginger, ground

Preparation:

Wash the apricots and cut into halves. Chop all into small pieces and set aside.

Rinse the Swiss chard thoroughly under cold running water. Drain and torn into small pieces. Set aside.

Peel the grapefruit and divide into wedges. Cut each wedge in half and set aside.

Wash the apple and cut lengthwise in half. Remove the core and chop into bite-sized pieces. Set aside.

Now, combine apricots, Swiss chard, grapefruit, and apple in a juicer and process until juiced. Transfer to a serving glass and stir in the honey and ginger.

Add few ice cubes and serve immediately.

Nutrition information per serving: Kcal: 212, Protein: 4.7g, Carbs: 61.9g, Fats: 1.1g

ADDITIONAL TITLES FROM THIS AUTHOR

70 Effective Meal Recipes to Prevent and Solve Being Overweight: Burn Fat Fast by Using Proper Dieting and Smart Nutrition

By

Joe Correa CSN

48 Acne Solving Meal Recipes: The Fast and Natural Path to Fixing Your Acne Problems in Less Than 10 Days!

By

Joe Correa CSN

41 Alzheimer's Preventing Meal Recipes: Reduce or Eliminate Your Alzheimer's Condition in 30 Days or Less!

By

Joe Correa CSN

70 Effective Breast Cancer Meal Recipes: Prevent and Fight Breast Cancer with Smart Nutrition and Powerful Foods

By

Joe Correa CSN